# My ADHD Life Journal

## Building Self-Awareness

# Meryl Bengtsson

# Acknowledgments

I would like to acknowledge Sharlene Page—my collaborative partner who truly supports me. The writing of this book would not have been possible without her countless edits, suggestions, typing, and counsel throughout the process.

# About the Author

From restlessness to discovery, Meryl Bengtsson's journey of ADHD self-awareness is a testament to resilience and growth. In this journal, she shares insights gleaned from years of crossing continents, nurturing a decades-long marriage, and navigating paths that didn't always go as planned.

Through focused reflection, she found clarity amid life's uncertainties. Now, she invites others to discover the calm, creativity, and purpose that unfold when embracing an ADHD mind.

Whether seeking a new perspective or a moment of peace, this journal offers a guiding light toward self-discovery.

# My ADHD Self-Awareness Journal!

We have designed this journal to support you in your ADHD journey, cultivating the practice of self-awareness. This encourages you to listen to your inner voice, learn from your behaviors, and leverage new strengths as you track your personal growth.

To kickstart your self-awareness journey, we have created a space to start dreaming, reflecting, and focusing on your strengths to better navigate your ADHD life.

The daily pages will guide you in tracking your ADHD life, acknowledging your emotions, and using sections designed to help you listen, learn, and leverage your journey. There is also space to explore your thoughts and ideas.

**ADHD Life Tip!**

How you view your challenges will determine how you process them into your zone of control.

*"ADHD Makes Life Paradoxical: You can super focus, but you can space out when you least mean to. You can radiate confidence and feel as insecure as a cat in a kennel. You can perform at the highest level while feeling incompetent as you do so. You can be loved by so many but feel as if no one really likes you. You can totally intend to do something, then forget to do it. You can have the greatest ideas in the world but feel as if you can't accomplish a thing."*

**—Dr. Edward M. Hallowell,**
**Psychiatrist and leading authority on ADHD, Harvard graduate**.

# How to Use This Journal

This ADHD Self-Awareness Journal is your personal space for exploring thoughts, emotions, and discoveries about how your mind works. Each section begins with a short introduction, followed by guided reflections designed to encourage insight and self-discovery. You'll find prompts that invite you to pause, observe, and jot down whatever comes to mind.

- **Start Where You Are:** Skim through the journal and begin with a reflection that resonates with you in the moment. There's no single "right" place to start—only the place that sparks your curiosity.

- **Engage with the Prompts:** Each prompt is crafted to help you notice patterns, feelings, and behaviors that might otherwise slip by. Use them to channel your creativity, vent frustrations, or brainstorm new ideas.

- **Write (or Sketch) Your Heart Out:** These pages are your canvas. There's no need for perfect spelling or grammar—your honest thoughts are more important than polished sentences.

- **Make It Your Own:** Feel free to add stickers, doodles, or any personal touches that make this journal feel like a reflection of you.

- **Reflect Often:** Revisit previous entries whenever you need reminders of your insights or a boost of motivation. Over time, you'll see how your perspectives evolve and deepen.

Above all, this journal is meant to be encouraging and enjoyable—a companion on your journey toward greater self-awareness and appreciation of your wonderfully unique ADHD mind. Let these reflections spark joy, curiosity, and acceptance as you track your growth day by day.

*"I'm not easily distracted; I'm just passionately curious about everything all at once."* **– Anonymous**

# My Story – Meryl Bengtsson

If I had to choose one word to describe my life, it would be **"restless."** In many ways, this restlessness has been a blessing—it led me to take risks that enriched my life, including moving to Denmark, meeting my husband (we've been married 37 years now!), and having our wonderful son.

Yet, the same restlessness has also acted as a saboteur, pushing me to move from country to country, job to job, house to house—often for the wrong reasons or with outcomes that didn't match my hopes. You get the picture!

Some might say being restless is simply part of growing up or building character. However, I noticed that many people around me didn't share this same urgency to uproot and start anew, and my own snap decisions sometimes set me back. Curious about why I felt so restless, I began reading about ADHD. The more I learned, the more I recognized myself in its descriptions.

I've come to see self-awareness as a crucial executive function. Yet, in our busy lives, we rarely pause to breathe, reflect, and truly notice our feelings and choices. Self-awareness and reflection open the door to growth—they help us shape our core values, beliefs, and mindset.

Journaling became my personal pathway to clarity, and it has brought me so much peace. I created this journal in the hope that you, too, will discover the joy and inner calm that come from taking a few moments each day to reconnect with yourself.

*"My mind doesn't wander aimlessly; it explores boundless possibilities with every leap."* **– Meryl Bengtsson**

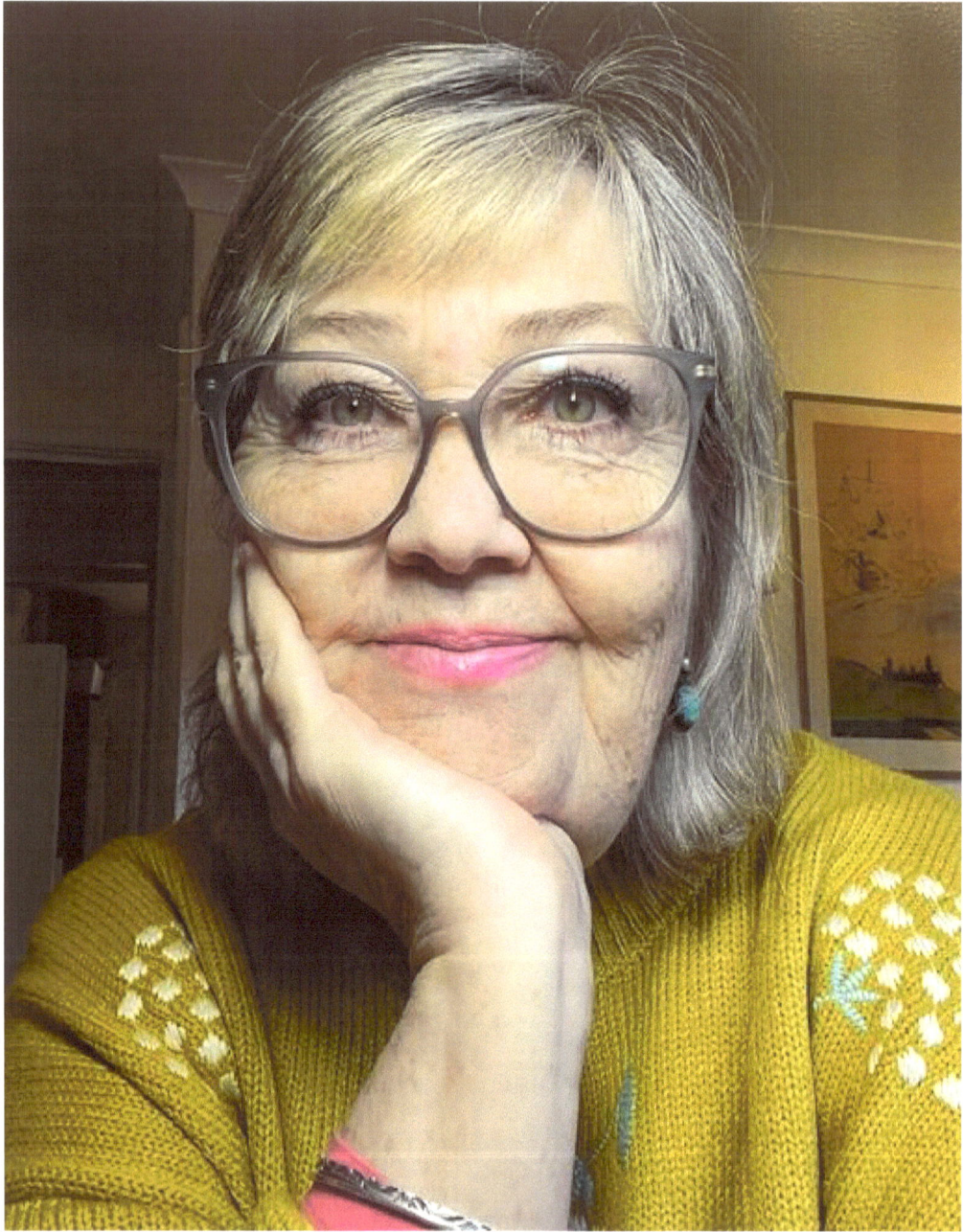

# ADHD Life Circle of Balance

Before you embark on your journaling journey, map out your Circle of Balance. This will help you focus on areas that need attention and track your progress!

As you move through these questions, pause where something feels heavy. Notice where you feel light. Let this be a starting point, not a judgment. This honest reflection isn't about fixing every part of your life—it's about recognizing what needs more care, attention, or understanding.

Take your time. Breathe into discomfort. Celebrate what's working. This is your space to listen, learn, and begin to truly know yourself.

**How to Use:**

- Read the three prompts under each category.
- Choose the response that feels most true for each statement.
- Add up your total score for the category.
- Mark your score on the provided Circle of Balance chart and connect your points.

**Scoring System:**

Each statement has three response options. Circle the one that resonates most with you.

☐ **1 Point** – This area is a challenge, and I struggle with it regularly.

☐ **2 Points** – This area is inconsistent—I have good and bad days.

☐ **3 Points** – This area feels stable, and I'm generally satisfied.

At the end of each category, add up your total score (out of 9) and record it in the space provided.

## 1. Physical Health & Energy *(Body, movement, sleep, vitality)*

- I wake up feeling rested and refreshed.

  ☐ Rarely (1) | ☐ Sometimes (2) | ☐ Often (3)

- My eating habits and hydration support my energy levels.

  ☐ Not at all (1) | ☐ Somewhat (2) | ☐ Yes, mostly (3)

- My body feels strong and capable rather than tense or sluggish.

  ☐ No (1) | ☐ Somewhat (2) | ☐ Yes (3)

**Total Score for Physical Health: ____ / 9**

## 2. Mental & Emotional Well-being *(Stress, mood, emotional balance)*

- I can recognize and process my emotions rather than suppressing or avoiding them.

  ☐ No (1) | ☐ Sometimes (2) | ☐ Yes (3)

- My thoughts feel supportive and encouraging rather than critical or overwhelming.

  ☐ No (1) | ☐ Sometimes (2) | ☐ Yes (3)

- I have strategies to manage stress and calm my mind when needed.

  ☐ No (1) | ☐ Sometimes (2) | ☐ Yes (3)

**Total Score for Mental & Emotional Well-being: ____ / 9**

## 3. Relationships & Connection *(Support, communication, social well-being)*

- I feel genuinely connected to at least one person who understands and supports me.

  ☐ No (1) | ☐ Sometimes (2) | ☐ Yes (3)

- My relationships energize rather than drain me.

  ☐ No (1) | ☐ Sometimes (2) | ☐ Yes (3)

- I show up authentically in my relationships rather than masking or people-pleasing.

  ☐ No (1) | ☐ Sometimes (2) | ☐ Yes (3)

**Total Score for Relationships & Connection: ____ / 9**

## 4. Work, Purpose & Responsibilities *(Career, tasks, motivation)*

- I feel a sense of purpose in my work or daily responsibilities.

  ☐ No (1) | ☐ Sometimes (2) | ☐ Yes (3)

- I can complete important tasks without constant procrastination or stress.

  ☐ No (1) | ☐ Sometimes (2) | ☐ Yes (3)

- I feel engaged and capable in my work rather than just surviving the day.

  ☐ No (1) | ☐ Sometimes (2) | ☐ Yes (3)

**Total Score for Work & Purpose:** _____ / 9

## 5. Environment & Surroundings *(Organization, comfort, space)*

- My environment supports my focus rather than distracting or overwhelming me.

  ☐ No (1) | ☐ Sometimes (2) | ☐ Yes (3)

- I have systems or routines that help keep my space functional.

  ☐ No (1) | ☐ Sometimes (2) | ☐ Yes (3)

- I feel comfortable and at ease in my surroundings.

  ☐ No (1) | ☐ Sometimes (2) | ☐ Yes (3)

**Total Score for Environment:** _____ / 9

## 6. Finances & Stability *(Money, security, financial habits)*

- I feel in control of my financial situation.

  ☐ No (1) | ☐ Sometimes (2) | ☐ Yes (3)

- I manage my finances with clarity and awareness rather than avoidance or stress.

  ☐ No (1) | ☐ Sometimes (2) | ☐ Yes (3)

- I make intentional financial decisions that align with my needs.

  ☐ No (1) | ☐ Sometimes (2) | ☐ Yes (3)

**Total Score for Finances & Stability:** _____ / 9

### 7. Self-Talk & Inner Dialogue *(Mindset, self-compassion, confidence)*

- My inner voice is mostly kind rather than critical or self-defeating.

  ☐ No (1) | ☐ Sometimes (2) | ☐ Yes (3)

- I recover quickly from setbacks rather than spiraling into self-doubt.

  ☐ No (1) | ☐ Sometimes (2) | ☐ Yes (3)

- I give myself grace and patience, especially when I struggle.

  ☐ No (1) | ☐ Sometimes (2) | ☐ Yes (3)

**Total Score for Self-Talk & Inner Dialogue: _____ / 9**

### 8. Hobbies, Joy & Creativity *(Passions, play, fulfillment)*

- I regularly engage in hobbies or activities that bring me joy.

  ☐ No (1) | ☐ Sometimes (2) | ☐ Yes (3)

- I prioritize fun and creativity rather than letting them be last on my list.

  ☐ No (1) | ☐ Sometimes (2) | ☐ Yes (3)

- I feel fulfilled by activities outside of work and responsibilities.

  ☐ No (1) | ☐ Sometimes (2) | ☐ Yes (3)

**Total Score for Hobbies & Joy: _____ / 9**

# Interpreting Your Circle of Balance

**Step 1: Add up your total score for all eight categories.**

**Final Total Score:** ____ / 72

*"Balance is not something you find; it's something you create."* – Jana Kingsford

**Step 2: Mark Each Category's Score on the Circle of Balance Chart**

- **0–3 points** → Inner circle (*Needs attention*)
- **4–6 points** → Middle circle (*Somewhat balanced*)
- **7–9 points** → Outer circle (*Thriving*)

**Step 3: Connect the Dots Across All Categories**

- A smooth, full circle suggests **good balance**.
- An uneven, jagged shape highlights **areas needing more care**.

**Step 4: Reflect on Your Balance**

- What areas feel strong?
- Where do you see gaps or struggles?
- What's one small step you could take to improve balance?

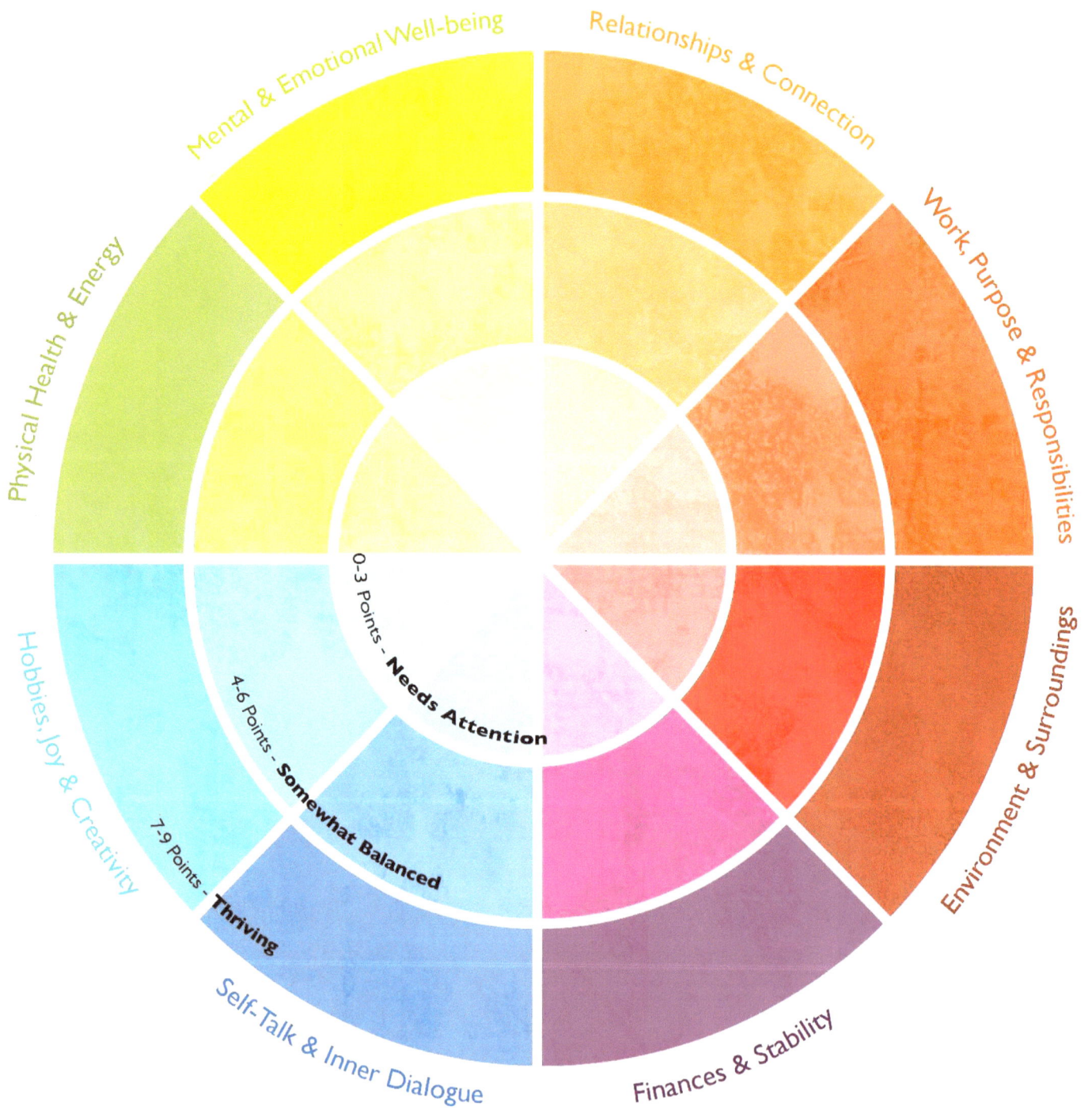

Mental & Emotional Well-being

Relationships & Connection

Physical Health & Energy

Work, Purpose & Responsibilities

Environment & Surroundings

Hobbies, Joy & Creativity

Finances & Stability

Self-Talk & Inner Dialogue

0-3 Points - **Needs Attention**

4-6 Points - **Somewhat Balanced**

7-9 Points - **Thriving**

# My ADHD Life Dreams

Listen to your soul, give yourself permission to dream big, and allow your thoughts to flow freely as you explore the possibilities of a limitless life!

**Live, Love & Laugh**

Describe it, insert pictures or doodle—there is no right or wrong way. This is your space—color your life outside the box!

This is your space to dream without limits—no rules, no pressure, just imagination running free. Scribble, sketch, or splash your ideas onto the page however they come to you.

- What if anything were possible?
- What would bring you the most joy?
- What makes you feel truly alive?

**Need Inspiration?**

Imagine waking up anywhere, trying something new, or living life exactly as you want.

*"Don't be pushed around by the fears in your mind. Be led by the dreams in your heart."* — **Roy T. Bennett**

# Living Your ADHD Life Dreams in 3D!

*e.g., "Knowledge – Find a course that interests me!"*

*"Your dreams are the architects of your destiny. Let them build a life that defies all limits."* — **Unknown**

# Loving Yourself & Your ADHD Life!

*e.g., "Self-Care – Journal daily!"*

*"To love oneself is the beginning of a lifelong romance."* — **Oscar Wilde**

# Laughing Your Way
# Through Your ADHD Life!

*e.g., "Friends – go on holiday together to celebrate our friendship!"*

*"Laughter is timeless, imagination has no age, and dreams are forever."* — **Walt Disney**

# The Big Dream in 3D

*"Your vision will become clear only when you can look into your own heart. Who looks outside, dreams; who looks inside, awakes."* — **Carl Jung**

16

**Loving ourselves through the process of owning our story is the bravest thing we will ever do.**

– Brené Brown

# My Personal Reflections

**Pause and Take a Breath**

You've taken time to explore your Circle of Balance—mapping out where things feel steady and where they might need more attention. You've also allowed yourself to dream, imagining the life you want to create.

Now, let's shift into reflection.

Before rushing into action, give yourself space to sit with what you've uncovered. Reflection is about noticing—without pressure, without judgment. It's about understanding the connections between your dreams and your current reality.

_____

_____

_____

_____

_____

_____

_____

_____

- **As I look at my Circle of Balance, what stands out?**

- **Do any areas feel more connected to my dreams than others?**

- **What emotions am I feeling as I reflect on my balance and dreams?**

# Why Reflection Matters

ADHD often makes it easy to move quickly from one thought to the next. Reflection helps slow things down and allows you to:

- **Notice Patterns** – Recognizing where your energy naturally flows and where you feel stuck.

- **Acknowledge What Feels Right** – Identifying the areas of life that already align with your vision.

- **Make Sense of Feelings** – Processing any frustration, excitement, or uncertainty.

- **Find Clarity** – Taking time to understand what's emerging before moving forward.

<br>

_____

_____

_____

_____

_____

_____

- **Do I see any differences between my dreams and my current balance?**

- **Are there areas where I already feel aligned?**

- **What surprises me about this reflection?**

*"Life can only be understood backwards, but it must be lived forwards."*
— **Søren Kierkegaard**

# Word Mapping

Sometimes a single word can hold a lot of meaning.

1. Choose one word that stood out to you as you explored your *Circle of Balance* and *ADHD Life Dreams*.

2. Write it in the center of the page.

3. Around it, jot down related thoughts, emotions, or situations that come to mind.

4. Let your mind explore connections freely—there are no wrong answers.

*"Not until we are lost do we begin to understand ourselves."* — **Henry David Thoreau**

# Sentence Starters

Use these prompts to unlock deeper thoughts that may be lingering beneath the surface.

**• One thing I didn't realize before is...**

_____

_____

_____

_____

**• When I think about my balance, I feel...**

_____

_____

_____

_____

**• If I could focus on one small shift right now, it would be...**

_____

_____

_____

_____

*"The greatest weapon against stress is our ability to choose one thought over another."* — **William James**

# Freewriting Moments

Let your thoughts flow without overthinking.

Set a timer for 5 minutes and write about the connection between your current reality and your dreams. No editing. No structure. Just words.

**Prompt:** *What do I understand better about myself after this exploration?*

_____

_____

_____

_____

_____

_____

_____

_____

_____

_____

_____

_____

_____

_____

*"Writing is an exploration. You start from nothing and learn as you go."*

— **E.L. Doctorow**

# Check-In Words

Pick three words that describe how you're feeling right now.

Reflect on why these words showed up.

**Example:** *Restless. Curious. Hopeful.*

- Why am I restless?

- What am I curious about?

- How can I nurture my hope?

Write your three words and explore their meaning.

| | | |
|---|---|---|
| | | |
| | | |
| | | |
| | | |
| | | |
| | | |
| | | |
| | | |
| | | |
| | | |

*"Fill your paper with the breathings of your heart."* — **William Wordsworth**

# Making Sense of What You've Discovered

Now that you've explored your current balance and your future dreams, take a moment to reflect.

**Observe Without Judgment**

- What themes or patterns are emerging?

_____
_____
_____

- Are there areas where your current balance already supports your dreams?

_____
_____
_____

- Are there areas that feel misaligned or need attention?

_____
_____
_____

**"One thing I noticed about my reflections is…"**

_____
_____
_____

_"Reflection is the lamp of the heart. If it departs, the heart will have no light."_

**— Abdullah ibn Alawi al-Haddad**

# Identify One Focus Area

It's tempting to want to change everything at once, but lasting change comes from small, intentional steps.

- Choose one area that feels most important to explore first.
- Ask yourself:
    - Why does this area stand out to me?
    - What would it feel like if it were more in balance?

**"The area I want to focus on first is… because…"**

_____
_____
_____
_____
_____
_____
_____
_____
_____
_____
_____

*"The journey of a thousand miles begins with one step."* — **Lao Tzu**

**Break It Down into Small, Gentle Steps**

Change happens through small, manageable shifts. ADHD can make big goals feel overwhelming, so let's focus on one small step.

**Examples:**

- If you want more balance in health, a small step could be drinking one extra glass of water today.

- If emotional well-being needs support, try pausing for five minutes of quiet.

- If relationships feel out of sync, consider sending a quick message to someone who matters to you.

"A small step I can take is…"

_____

_____

_____

_____

_____

_____

_____

_____

_____

_____

_____

_____

*"The secret of getting ahead is getting started."* — **Mark Twain**

# My ADHD Life Today Tracker

**How are you feeling today?**

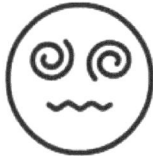

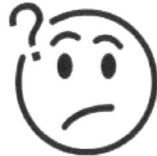

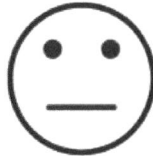

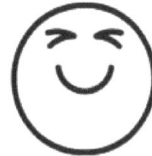

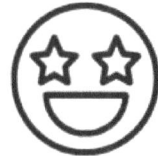

_____

_____

_____

_____

_____

_____

_____

_____

_____

_____

_____

_____

_____

_____

# How are you feeling today?

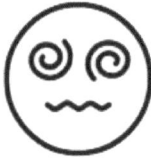

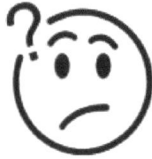

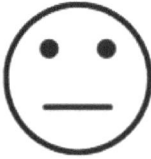

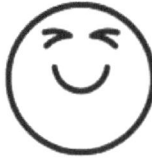

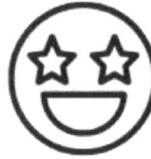

# How are you feeling today?

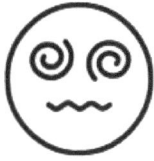

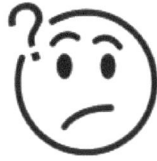

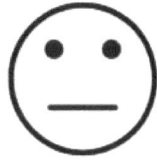

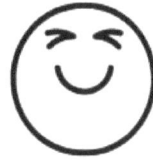

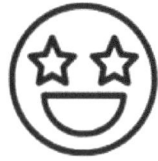

# How are you feeling today?

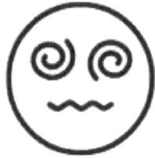

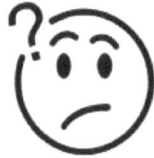

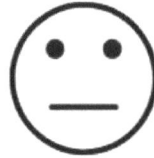

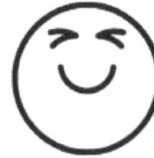

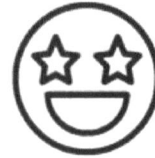

# How are you feeling today?

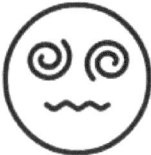

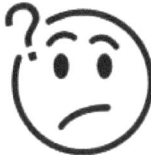

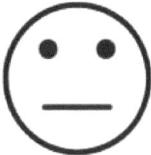

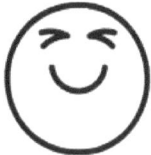

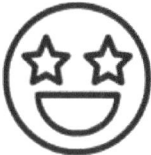

# How are you feeling today?

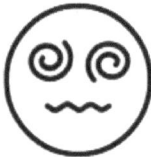

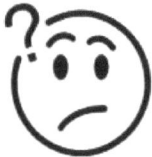

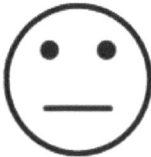

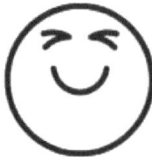

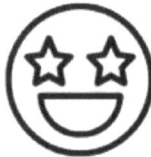

# How are you feeling today?

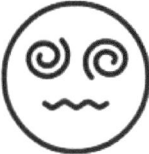

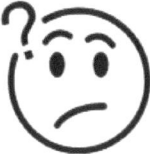

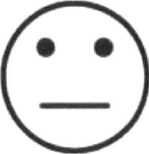

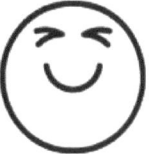

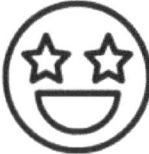

_____
_____
_____
_____
_____
_____
_____
_____
_____
_____
_____
_____
_____
_____

# Start Your Day with Intention

Each day, take a moment to pause, check in with yourself, and set the tone for the day ahead. This journal is your space to listen, learn, and leverage—guiding you toward a more balanced ADHD life.

**Creative Space**

Before diving into your journaling, take a moment to express yourself freely. Use this space to:

- Doodle, draw, or scribble whatever comes to mind.

- Paste pictures, stickers, or anything that inspires you.

- Jot down a thought, quote, or random idea floating in your mind.

# Listening: Tuning into Your Inner Voice

- What is my inner voice telling me today?

_____

_____

_____

_____

_____

- What thoughts, emotions, or sensations am I noticing?

_____

_____

_____

_____

_____

- What do I need to acknowledge or be aware of?

_____

_____

_____

_____

_____

# Learning:
# Recognizing Patterns and Insights

- What am I learning about myself today?

_____
_____
_____
_____
_____

- Did I notice anything about my energy, focus, or emotions?

_____
_____
_____
_____
_____

- Are there any repeating thoughts or challenges I should explore?

_____
_____
_____
_____
_____

# Leveraging:

# Taking Small, Intentional Steps

- How can I use what I know to support myself today?

_____
_____
_____
_____
_____

- What small action can I take that aligns with my needs?

_____
_____
_____
_____
_____

- How can I lean into my strengths?

_____
_____
_____
_____
_____

# Noticing and Navigating

Growth isn't about getting everything right every time—it's about paying attention to what works, what doesn't, and adjusting with self-awareness.

- What felt good today, and why?

_____

_____

_____

_____

_____

- What didn't go as planned, and what might I try differently tomorrow?

_____

_____

_____

_____

_____

- What small shift could help me navigate tomorrow with more ease?

_____

_____

_____

_____

_____

# Celebrating My Wins

**What's one thing I did well today, no matter how small?**

- A moment of kindness, a task completed, a challenge faced—every win counts!

- Let yourself express it visually—doodle, sketch, scribble, or add anything that feels like a win today.

Mindfulness
is the practice of
bringing one's attention
to the present moment,
without judgement.

– Jon Kabat-Zinn

# Weekly Moment Check-In

## Body Scan: Tuning Into How You Feel

Pause. Breathe. Take a quiet moment to check in with your body.

Start at your toes and slowly move upward, noticing any sensations. Where do you feel tension? Where do you feel lightness?

No need to change anything—just observe.

Let this be a space to connect with how you feel, right here, right now.

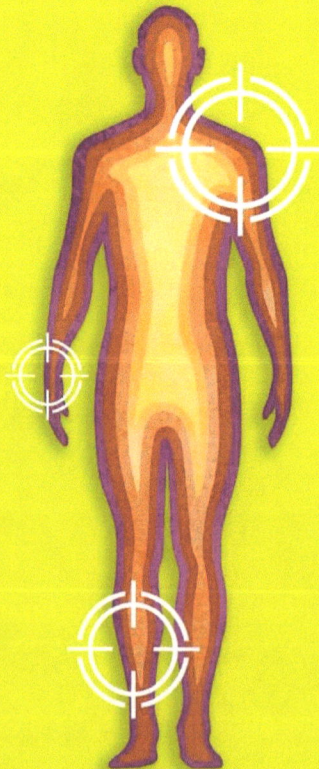

# Body Scan: Tuning Into How You Feel

Pause. Breathe. Take a quiet moment to check in with your body.

Start at your toes and slowly move upward, noticing any sensations. Where do you feel tension? Where do you feel lightness?

No need to change anything—just observe.

Let this be a space to connect with how you feel, right here, right now.

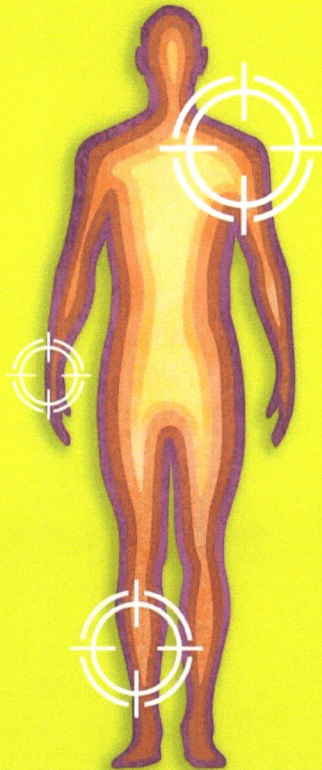

# Body Scan: Tuning Into How You Feel

Pause. Breathe. Take a quiet moment to check in with your body.

Start at your toes and slowly move upward, noticing any sensations. Where do you feel tension? Where do you feel lightness?

No need to change anything—just observe.

Let this be a space to connect with how you feel, right here, right now.

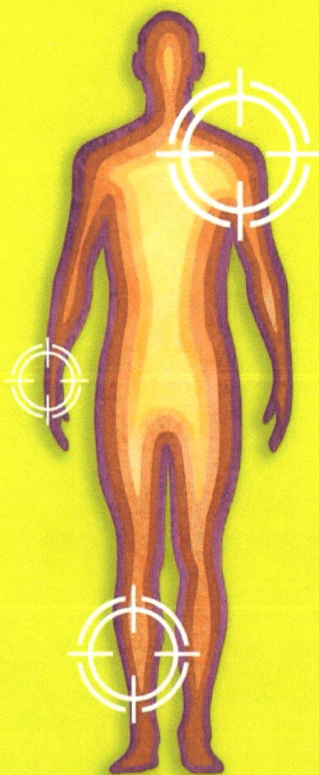

# Body Scan: Tuning Into How You Feel

Pause. Breathe. Take a quiet moment to check in with your body.

Start at your toes and slowly move upward, noticing any sensations. Where do you feel tension? Where do you feel lightness?

No need to change anything—just observe.

Let this be a space to connect with how you feel, right here, right now.

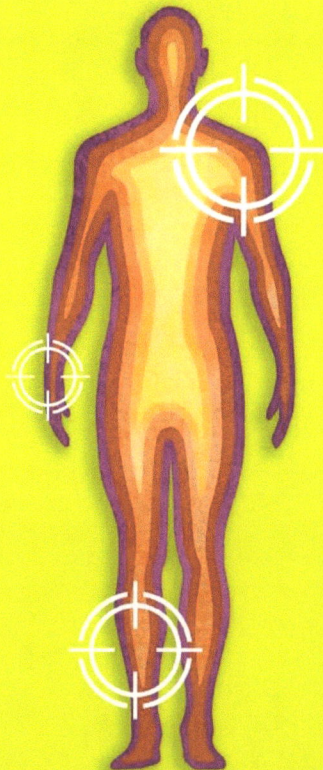

# Body Scan: Tuning Into How You Feel

Pause. Breathe. Take a quiet moment to check in with your body.

Start at your toes and slowly move upward, noticing any sensations. Where do you feel tension? Where do you feel lightness?

No need to change anything—just observe.

Let this be a space to connect with how you feel, right here, right now.

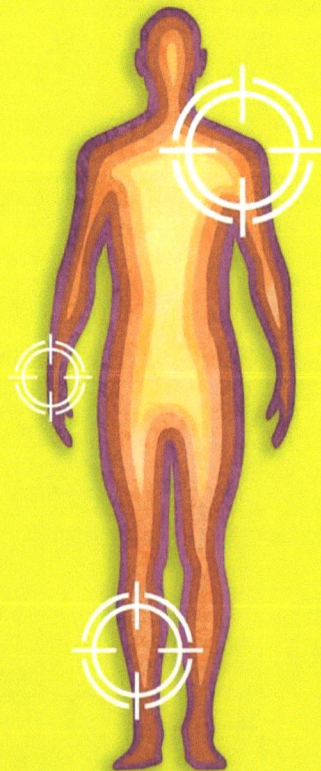

# Body Scan: Tuning Into How You Feel

Pause. Breathe. Take a quiet moment to check in with your body.

Start at your toes and slowly move upward, noticing any sensations. Where do you feel tension? Where do you feel lightness?

No need to change anything—just observe.

Let this be a space to connect with how you feel, right here, right now.

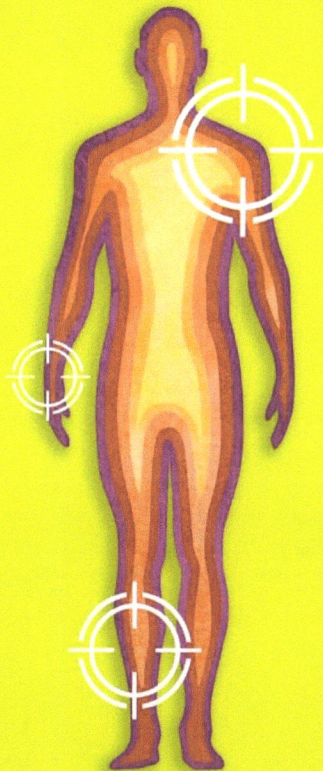

# Body Scan: Tuning Into How You Feel

Pause. Breathe. Take a quiet moment to check in with your body.

Start at your toes and slowly move upward, noticing any sensations. Where do you feel tension? Where do you feel lightness?

No need to change anything—just observe.

Let this be a space to connect with how you feel, right here, right now.

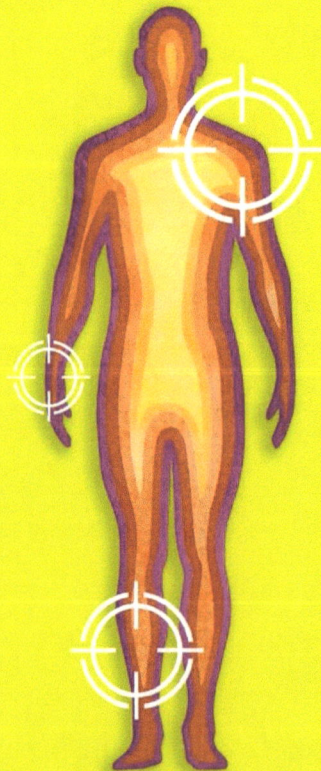

# Discover Your ADHD Prowess

- What strengths have shown up for you this week?

- Maybe it was your creativity in problem-solving, your ability to think fast and adapt, or the way you hyper-focused and brought something to life. Or maybe it was simply your resilience—getting through a tough moment.

- Jot down the ADHD strengths you've discovered or embraced this week.

|  |  |  |
|---|---|---|
|  |  |  |
|  |  |  |

_____

_____

_____

_____

_____

_____

_____

_____

_____

*"Your ADHD is a part of you, but it doesn't define you. Embrace your unique brain, and let it be the source of your strength and creativity."* – **Dr. Edward Hallowell**

# Monthly Moment Check-In

You've been journaling for a while now—capturing thoughts, exploring feelings, and noticing patterns. Before continuing, let's pause and reflect.

Not to measure success. Not to judge. Just to see where you are now.

Look back at your Circle of Balance, your Dreams, and your Journey. What's shifted? What's still unfolding? What feels different?

*"Success is not the key to happiness. Happiness is the key to success. If you love what you are doing, you will be successful."* – **Albert Schweitzer**

# Monthly Moment Check-In

You've been journaling for a while now—capturing thoughts, exploring feelings, and noticing patterns. Before continuing, let's pause and reflect.

Not to measure success. Not to judge. Just to see where you are now.

Look back at your Circle of Balance, your Dreams, and your Journey. What's shifted? What's still unfolding? What feels different?

# Monthly Moment Check-In

You've been journaling for a while now—capturing thoughts, exploring feelings, and noticing patterns. Before continuing, let's pause and reflect.

Not to measure success. Not to judge. Just to see where you are now.

Look back at your Circle of Balance, your Dreams, and your Journey. What's shifted? What's still unfolding? What feels different?

# Where Am I Now?

Flip back to the last time you mapped your Circle of Balance.

There's no right or wrong—just take note.

- What has changed, even in small ways?

> _____
>
> _____
>
> _____
>
> _____

- Are there areas that feel lighter, easier, or clearer?

> _____
>
> _____
>
> _____
>
> _____

- Are there places where you still feel stuck?

> _____
>
> _____
>
> _____
>
> _____

*"Happiness lies in the joy of achievement and the thrill of creative effort."*

**– Franklin D. Roosevelt**

# Catching Up with My Dreams

Dreams aren't meant to stay still. They grow, shift, and sometimes, surprise us.

- Have any of my dreams taken a small step forward?

_____
_____
_____
_____
_____

- Are there new dreams I want to add?

_____
_____
_____
_____
_____

- Do any of my original dreams feel different now?

_____
_____
_____
_____
_____

# Write freely. No pressure. Just an open space to notice.

_"The future belongs to those who believe in the beauty of their dreams."_

**– Eleanor Roosevelt**

# Noticing the Patterns

Life speaks to us in patterns—sometimes whispers, sometimes echoes.

- What keeps coming up in my journal entries?

_____
_____
_____
_____
_____

- Are there any themes in how I feel, think, or act?

_____
_____
_____
_____
_____

- Have I surprised myself with anything I've written?

_____
_____
_____
_____
_____

# Let this space be for curiosity, not conclusions.

# What Feels Important Right Now?

**As you move forward, what feels like it deserves more attention?**

- Is there one small shift I'd like to explore?

_____
_____
_____
_____
_____

- A feeling I want to understand better?

_____
_____
_____
_____
_____

- A dream I'm ready to lean into?

_____
_____
_____
_____
_____

**Trust what comes up.**

**Let it be your quiet guide for the next stretch of journaling.**

Your self-discovery doesn't need to be loud or grandiose. It just needs to be **HONEST.**

– Unknown

# Keep Going—Your Journey Is Unfolding

This isn't the end. It's a pause. A moment to recognize how far you've come before stepping forward again.

Through these pages, you've listened to yourself, explored your patterns, and mapped out dreams that matter to you. Some days may have felt clear, others uncertain—but every time you showed up here, you were building something important: awareness, understanding, and trust in yourself.

Your ADHD journey is always evolving. Keep journaling, keep reflecting, and most importantly—keep moving in the direction that feels right for you.

- What's one thing I've learned about myself through this journal?

_____

_____

_____

_____

_____

- What's one small piece of advice I'd give my future self?

_____

_____

_____

_____

_____

If you're looking for deeper support, **ADHD Life** offers community, courses, and coaching to help you navigate your next steps. Whether you want to connect with others, explore new strategies, or work one-on-one with a coach, you don't have to do this alone.

Find more at www.adhdlife.works

When you're ready, start a new journal. Keep writing your story. You're already on the path—just keep going.

*"The journey of self-discovery with ADHD is not about perfection but about progress, understanding, and self-compassion."*

**– Dr. Edward Hallowell, ADHD Expert and Author**

www.ingramcontent.com/pod-product-compliance
Lightning Source LLC
Chambersburg PA
CBHW061140030426
42335CB00002B/58